SCOLIOSIS CURE MANUAL

The Absolute step by step guide on the best treatment for scoliosis

By

Dr. Harvey Donald

Copyright @ 2023

Table of Contents

PREFACE

This book will certainly guide you on everything you ought to know and completely understand about scoliosis and its treatment. The book will guide you on the types and forms of scoliosis, symptoms and signs of scoliosis, causes and risk factors, complications, diagnosis and tests for scoliosis, treatment and prevention, natural home remedies, scoliosis recommended diet, exercises and stretching exercises for scoliosis and so much more.

CHAPTER ONE

INTRODUCTION

Scoliosis which is most usually diagnosed in adolescents is a sideway curvature or an abnormal lateral curvature of the spine (backbone). There is a natural forward-and-backward curve to the spine or a sideways C- or S-shaped curve in the spine. With scoliosis, there is a spinal rotation along with a development of a side-to-side curve of the spine.

The **normal curves** of the spine occur at the *cervical, thoracic and lumbar regions* in the supposed *"sagittal"* plane.

Spinal curves are sometimes classified as **structural or nonstructural** by physicians. A structural curve is permanent and may be as a result of a medical condition or injury while a nonstructural curve is temporary, which entails that the spine is structurally normal. In either way, a physician will try to find and correct or treat the cause.

Scoliosis is often discovered during growth in childhood or adolescence (pediatric scoliosis), although when it starts or is found after puberty, it is referred to as "adult scoliosis".

Infantile scoliosis *can affect individuals before the age of 3 years, despite the fact that scoliosis is uncommon in infants.*

Scoliosis is usually described as spinal curvature in the *"coronal"* (frontal) plane and while the degree of curvature is measured on the coronal plane, scoliosis is literally a more complex, three-dimensional issue involving the following planes

(a) **Coronal plane-** The *coronal plane* is a vertical plane from head to foot and parallel to the shoulders, dissecting the body into anterior and posterior sections.

(b) **Axial plane/cardinal plane-** Lateral to the plane of the ground at right angles to the coronal and sagittal planes

(c) **Sagittal plane-** Divides the body into right and left halves.

Scoliosis affects about 2 to 3% of the population, or an estimated six to nine million individuals in the United States of America. Scoliosis can develop in infancy or early childhood, although the primary age of onset for scoliosis is around 10 to 15 years old, occurring uniformly among the female and male genders. Nevertheless, Females are more likely to progress to a curve magnitude that requires urgent treatment. Each year, scoliosis patients make more than 600,000 visits to private physician offices, with an estimated 30,000 children fitted with a brace and an estimated 38,000 patients undergoing spinal fusion surgery.

*In spite of the fact that scoliosis can occur in individuals with conditions such as **muscular dystrophy, spina bifida, and cerebral palsy,** the cause of the most childhood scoliosis is not known and this is referred to as **Idiopathic scoliosis.***

Most cases of scoliosis are mild, although some curves exacerbate as children grow. Severe scoliosis can be disabling and a particularly severe spinal curve can decrease the amount of space within the chest, thus making it hard for the lungs to function appropriately.

Children who have mild scoliosis are observed closely, often with X-rays, to see if the curve is getting aggravated. In numerous cases, no treatment is required. Some children may be required to wear a brace to stop the curve from getting worse while others may require surgery to straighten severe curves.

Furthermore, in adult, the degree of the spine curve may or may not ascertain treatment. Treatment is geared towards relieving symptoms, and not naturally fixing the curve. The aim is always to reduce pain and enhance function.

Despite the fact that scoliosis itself is painless; the normal age-related degeneration of the spine may result into symptoms and these symptoms are treated the same whether there is scoliosis or not. Scoliosis only becomes a factor when surgery is being suggested.

*Generally, most **scoliosis in adolescents** occurs in the thoracic or rib cage portion of the spine and in adults,* *the primary concern is basically in the lumbar or lower spine. The part or portion of the spine is most prone to changes seen with aging or degeneration.*

Note- *An abnormally rounded upper back greater than 50° of curvature is referred to as* **kyphosis.**

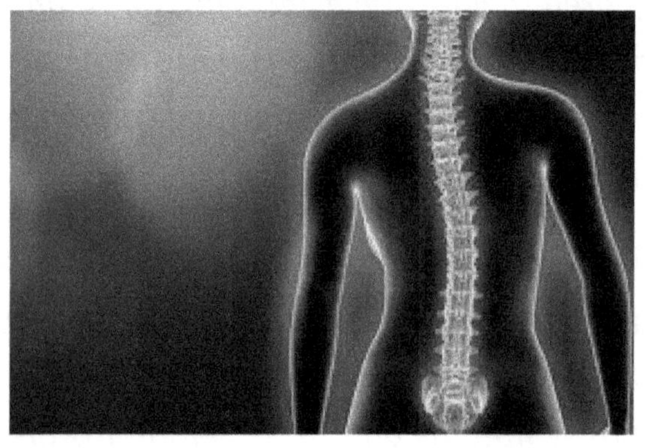

CHAPTER TWO

TYPES AND FORMS OF SCOLIOSIS

Scoliosis is any abnormal sideways curvature of the spine or backbone measuring at least 10° on an x-ray. Despite the fact that scoliosis is not a disease, in uncommon cases it can be caused by a disease.

Scoliosis can be broadly categorized into two and they include:

(a) **Structural scoliosis-** This is by far the most common category of scoliosis and it involves spinal rotation along with the side-to-side curvature of the spine or backbone. This ***structural scoliosis*** affects the spine's structure and is regarded permanent unless the spine or backbone receives treatment.

(b) **Nonstructural scoliosis-** Also known as *functional scoliosis,* this occurs from temporary cause and only involves a side-to-side curvature of the spine with the structure of the spine remaining normal. Causes of nonstructural scoliosis may include

- Having one leg longer than the other
- Muscle spasms, and some other types of *inflammation* such as *appendicitis.*

Nonstructural scoliosis is reversible and treating the underlying cause of scoliosis usually resolves the scoliosis.

If an individual with nonstructural scoliosis were to bend forward or lay down, the scoliosis curve would probably go away while held in that position.

Structural scoliosis is generally regarded more severe since it does not straighten out on its own and can possibly result in more spinal deformity.

There are various types of **Structural Scoliosis** and they include:

(a) **Idiopathic Scoliosis-** The idiopathic scoliosis which is the most common type of structural scoliosis accounts for around 8 to 10 cases of scoliosis and this type of scoliosis generally presents during adolescence, although it can also begin earlier in childhood or infancy. Currently, the cause of idiopathic scoliosis is unknown, although some research suggests genetics plays a part, but other factors are also probably involved to continue to be studied. Individuals with idiopathic scoliosis are usually diagnosed on routine physical examinations.

Furthermore, some individuals are diagnosed during health screenings performed in school settings.

Some individuals experience symptoms from scoliosis, and these symptoms bring the patient to medical attention. Idiopathic scoliosis is grouped by the age of the individual at the time of diagnosis.

Due to the alterations in shape and size of the thorax, idiopathic scoliosis may impact pulmonary function and present reports on pulmonary function testing in patients with mild to moderate idiopathic scoliosis demonstrated diminished pulmonary function.

- **Adolescent idiopathic scoliosis** is analyzed or diagnosed when a child or the patient is between the ages of 10 and 18 years. This phase covers the puberty stage and carries with it the largest risk of progression. The adolescent idiopathic scoliosis which affects about 4 to 5% of adolescents is more common in females, and while the reasons are not completely understood, a commonly accepted theory is that it is do with postural maturity.
- **Juvenile idiopathic Scoliosis** is analyzed or diagnosed when the

patient is between the ages of 4 and 9.

- **Infantile idiopathic Scoliosis** is diagnosed or analyzed when the patient is 3 years old or younger.
- **Adult idiopathic scoliosis** is diagnosed or analyzed when the patient is 18 years old and above. Although they can develop, cases of adult idiopathic scoliosis are not too common. In most cases, they are extensions of adolescent idiopathic scoliosis cases that went undiagnosed.

Understanding multifactorial causation is a vital aspect of understanding the nature of idiopathic conditions and when a condition is described as idiopathic, the condition's development can't be tied down to one single particular cause. Incidentally, an idiopathic condition can't have numerous causes; this is regarded as **multifactorial causation.**

When it comes to idiopathic scoliosis, it is typically accepted that it probably develops as a result of a combination of variables and that those variables can differ from patient to patient. From likely genetic imbalances, it is unknown which variables causes the development of abnormal spinal curvatures.

(b) **Neuromuscular Scoliosis-** The neuromuscular scoliosis which typically progresses more rapidly than idiopathic scoliosis and usually requires surgical treatment sometimes develops in individuals who are unable to walk as a result of a neuromuscular condition such as *cerebral palsy, marfan syndrome, spina bifida, or muscular dystrophy* and this type of scoliosis may also be referred to as **myopathic scoliosis.** It is a type of scoliosis that develops in children with medical conditions that impede the body's ability to control the muscles supporting the spine or backbone. In most instances of neuromuscular scoliosis, the scoliosis that develops is secondary to the other medical conditions the patient has.

- **Cerebral palsy-** Cerebral palsy is a condition identified by impaired muscle coordination and in numerous cases, cerebral palsy develops in children as a result of brain damage that occurred prior to during delivery.

Children with cerebral palsy have remarkably higher chances of developing scoliosis. They are most probably to develop the condition during their early years and into adolescence. The intensity of the scoliosis is closely connected or associated to the severity of cerebral palsy and can advance beyond skeletal maturity.

- **Spina bifida-** The spina bifida which can result into paralysis of the lower limbs and can also affect mental function is a congenital spinal defect where a gap in the spine or backbone exposes part of the spinal cord and its meninges.

Around 50% of individuals with spina bifida will develop scoliosis. Children with spina bifida at an increased risk for rapid progression and large spinal curvatures and these patients are observed closely to look out for progression during growth spurts.

- **Muscular dystrophy-** Muscular dystrophy is an uncommon progressive disease that affects voluntary muscles that control movement of the *legs,* trunk, and arms. Scoliosis is a common problem for individuals with **_muscular dystrophy._**

- **Marfan syndrome-** The marfan syndrome which commonly affects tall and thin individuals with long limbs is understood as a genetic disorder of the body's connective tissue. An estimated six out of ten individuals with **_marfan_** also have scoliosis and while the scoliosis that can develop with marfan syndrome is not generally severe, a growth spurt in a child with **_marfan syndrome_** can cause the scoliosis to progress.

(c) Congenital Scoliosis- The congenital scoliosis develops in utero and it is present in infancy. In these instances, there is a bone malformation that can cause a scoliosis to develop. Congenital scoliosis may occur in any location of the spine. Congenital scoliosis is often detected at a younger age than idiopathic scoliosis.

There is a known elevated incidence of other congenital abnormalities in children with congenital scoliosis, and these are mostly linked with the spinal cord, the heart, and the genitourinary system. When congenital scoliosis is diagnosed, it is vital that evaluation or assessment of the neurological, genitourinary and cardiovascular systems is undertaken.

An uncommon condition, affecting 1 in 10,000, it can result from malformations in the vertebrae or other causes and in most cases or instances, the spinal curve must be surgically corrected.

Other types of scoliosis may include:

(a) **Degenerative scoliosis-** This type of scoliosis occurs in older people (65 years and older) whose spinal discs are deteriorating as a result of the natural effects of aging, and this can result into the development of an abnormal spinal curvature. Degenerative scoliosis occurs most regularly in the lumbar spine (lower back). It is usually followed by spinal stenosis, or narrowing of the spinal canal, which compresses the spinal nerves and makes it hard for them to function properly. Back pain related with degenerative scoliosis often starts slowly and is connected with activity. The curvature of the spine in this form of scoliosis is usually relatively minor, and thus surgery may only be advised when conservative methods fail to relieve pain related with the condition.

(b) Traumatic scoliosis- Despite the fact that experts are not sure of how severe trauma has to be to cause the development of the condition, accidents can result into spinal deformities to develop.

(c) Syndromic scoliosis

(d) Scheuermann's kyphosis

CHAPTER THREE

SIGNS AND SYMPTOMS OF SCOLIOSIS

Scoliosis which often becomes noticeable from infancy or adolescence may lead to *low back pain, back stiffness, poor posture complications, joint and hip pain, fatigue, pain and numbness in the legs, difficulty in breathing as a result of the upper spine curve and fatigue as a result of muscle strain.*

The symptoms of scoliosis vary depending on the age of the individual.

Symptoms of scoliosis in adolescents

The most prevalent form of scoliosis appears in adolescence and it is referred to as ***adolescent***

idiopathic scoliosis. It can affect individuals between the ages of 10 and 18 years.

Some of the symptoms may include:

(a) The head appearing a bit off center or not centered directly above the pelvis.
(b) One hip appearing more prominent or higher than the other.
(c) Texture or appearance of the skin overlying the spine changes (hairy patches, dimples, and abnormalities in color).
(d) Uneven waist
(e) The ribs on each side as well as legs are of slightly different heights and slightly different lengths respectively.
(f) One side of the rib cage protruding forward.

(g) Clothes not hanging evenly and uniformly or not fitting properly.

(h) A rotating spine

(i) One shoulder or shoulder blade being higher or appearing prominent than the other

(j) uneven shoulders

(k) Individual leaning to one side as well as a prominence on one side of the back when bending forward.

Some types of scoliosis can result into back pain, although it is not often very painful. This symptom is more prevalent in older adults.

Symptoms of scoliosis in infants

Symptoms of scoliosis in infants may include:

(a) Persistently lying with the body curved to one side

(b) A lump on one side of the chest.

(c) In intense cases, problems with the heart and lungs, resulting to a shortness of breath and pain in the chest.

If an infant does not receive treatment for scoliosis, they will be more at risk of problems subsequently in life, such as lung function and impaired heart.

Symptoms of scoliosis in Adults

Most cases of adult scoliosis don't result into symptoms, although pain may develop. **Back pain** occurs for numerous reasons including arthritis, lack of ability to stand upright, and/as a result of weakness of the core musculature and loss of conditioning. If there is pressure on the nerves in the lumbar spine, leg pain, numbness or weakness may develop.

In some instances, body changes may include:

(a) Loss of height
(b) Irregular alignment of the hips and pelvis.

CHAPTER FOUR

CAUSES AND RISK FACTORS OF SCOLIOSIS

Physicians don't know what causes the most common form of scoliosis **(idiopathic scoliosis),** although it appears to involve hereditary factors, since the disorder sometimes runs in families.

Idiopathic scoliosis cannot be prevented and is not thought to be associated to things such as *exercise, diet or bad posture.*

Less common form of scoliosis may be caused by:

(a) Certain neuromuscular conditions such as *cerebral palsy, marfan syndrome, spinal cord trauma, spinal muscular atrophy, spina bifida, or muscular dystrophy.*

(b) Defects in birth which in turn affects the development of the bones of the spine.

(c) Infections of or injuries to the spine

(d) Wear and tear of the spine with age.

(e) Abnormalities of the spinal cord

(f) Initial or previous surgery on the chest wall as a baby.

(g) Tumor

Scoliosis Risk Factors

Some of the risk factors for developing the most common form of scoliosis may include:

(a) **Family History-** Having a family history with direct relatives affected by the scoliosis elevates an individual's chance of developing scoliosis. Nevertheless, most children with scoliosis don't have a family history of the condition.

(b) Age- Signs and symptoms tend to begin during a child's growth spurt which occurs just before puberty (basically between the ages of 9 and 15). Nevertheless, on the general perspective, symptoms start in adolescence.

(c) Sex- While both males and females develop mild scoliosis at around the same rate, the females have a much elevated risk of the curve aggravating and requiring more aggressive treatment.

CHAPTER FIVE

COMPLICATIONS OF SCOLIOSIS

Despite the fact that most individuals with scoliosis have a mild form of the disorder with relatively few adverse effects, scoliosis may occasionally cause certain complications such as:

(a) **Back problems/issues-** Individuals who had scoliosis as children may be more likely to develop chronic back pain, particularly if their abnormal curves are big and untreated.

(b) **Breathing difficulties-** In severe cases of scoliosis, the rib cage may press against the heart and lungs. This makes it hard to breathe and for the heart to pump, thus impairing the lungs and heart.

(c) Appearance- As scoliosis aggravates, it can result into more visible changes such as uneven hips and shoulders, prominent ribs, and a shift of the waist and trunk to one side. People with scoliosis usually become self-conscious about their appearance.

(d) Consistent pain particularly if there is wear and tear of the bones of the spine

(e) Leakage of spinal fluid as well as spinal infection after surgery

(f) Nerve damage from an uncorrected spinal surgery

*Scoliosis have been connected to **osteopenia** which is a condition that is marked by a loss of bone mass that causes bone density being lower than normal. Some physicians recommend that a bone density test be performed if an individual has scoliosis. Ascertaining* *the degree of bone loss may help in predicting the severity of spinal curvature progression.*

Furthermore, if osteopenia is left untreated, it may develop and progress into **osteoporosis** *which is a condition that affects the density of the bones and causes more severe loss of bone, eventually leading to brittle bones that easily fracture. The disease is commonly seen in postmenopausal women and adolescents with scoliosis have an increased risk of developing osteoporosis subsequently in their life.*

CHAPTER SIX

DIAGNOSIS AND TESTS FOR SCOLIOSIS

A physician will conduct a physical examination of the spine, shoulders, ribs, as well as the hips. With the help of a tool referred to as *inclinometer, or scoliometer,* the physician can measure the degree of scoliosis and an angle higher than 10° indicates scoliosis.

The curve is measured by the **Cobb method** and a positive diagnosis of scoliosis is performed based on a coronal curvature measured on a posterior-anterior radiograph of higher than 10°. Generally, a curve is considered significant if it is higher than 25° to 30°. Curves exceeding 45° to 50° are considered severe and usually require more aggressive treatment. The **Adam's Forward Bend Test** in which the patient leans forward with his or her feet together and bends 90° at the waist is a simple initial screening test that can detect potential problems, although cannot ascertain the precise type or severity of the deformity. Radiographic tests are needed for a precise and positive diagnosis.

Imaging scans including CT (Computerized tomography) scans, MRI (Magnetic resonance imaging) scans, and X-rays can help the physician to evaluate the shape, direction, location, and angle of the curve.

Furthermore, the physician may refer the individual to an orthopedic specialist for additional advice.

PHYSICAL EXAMINATION- Your physician will observe your back while you stand with your arms at your sides and will also check for spine curvature and whether your shoulders and waist area are equal.

Furthermore, your physician will ask you to bend forward, checking for any curvature in your upper and lower back.

Furthermore, neurological exam may also be conducted to check for numbness, abnormal reflexes, and muscle weakness.

IMAGING TESTS- Some of the imaging tests your physician may order to look for scoliosis may include:

(a) **MRI scan-** The MRI (Magnetic resonance imaging) scan uses radio and magnetic waves to get a clear image of bones and tissues surrounding them. A diagnostic test that creates 3-dimensional images of body structures using powerful magnets and computer technology; can reveal the spinal cord, nerve roots and surrounding areas as well as enlargement, degeneration and deformities.

(b) **X-ray-** During the X-ray test, *small amounts of radiation* are used in producing an image of your spine or backbone. Application of radiation to create a film or image of a part of the body can reveal the structure of the vertebrae and the outline of the joints.

(c) **CT scan-** During the CT (Computerized tomography) scan, *X-rays is taken at a range of angles* to acquire a 3-dimensional picture of the body. A diagnostic image or picture produced after a computer reads X-rays; can reveal the shape and size of the spinal canal, its contents and the structures around it. Very excellent at visualizing bony structures.

(d) Bone scan- The bone scan test detects a radioactive solution injected into your blood that concentrates in areas of elevated circulation, identifying *spinal abnormalities.*

(e) Ultrasound

Adult scoliosis diagnosis

Scoliosis that occurs or is diagnosed in adulthood is distinguishable from childhood scoliosis, since the primary causes and aims of treatment differ in patients who have already attained skeletal maturity. Most adults with scoliosis can be divided into the following group:

- Adult scoliosis patients who were originally surgically treated as adolescents

- Adults who did not receive treatment when they were younger as well as adults with a form or type of scoliosis referred to as **degenerative scoliosis.**

A medical history is normally taken for adult scoliosis prior to treatment and you may be asked questions such as:

(a) The date you first observed a change in your spine
(b) Family history
(c) Curve progression (ascertained from initial X-rays, if accessible)
(d) Presence and location of pain

Your nerves may be tested via reflex, sensation and muscle-strength checks. In adults with scoliosis, X-rays are often suggested once in every five years, unless symptoms are getting progressively aggravated.

CHAPTER SEVEN

TREATMENT OF SCOLIOSIS

The treatment of scoliosis varies, and this depends on the severity of the curve. Children who have very mild curve often don't require any treatment at all, but they may require frequent checkups to see if the curve is aggravating as they grow. With a curve of 10° to 25°, a physician will often have checkups with the individual at 3, 6 or 12 month intervals to check if the condition is changing.

For a 40° curve, a physician may suggest bracing and if the curve is higher than this, surgery may be recommended.

The majority of cases of adult scoliosis can be managed non-operatively via frequent observation by a physician, over-the-counter medications, as well as core-strengthening exercises to strengthen your back and abdomen and also to enhance flexibility. If you smoke, it is vital you stop smoking as smoking has been shown to quicken degenerative process.

In most instances, your physician will suggest or recommend some forms of physical therapy, to both maintain strength and ease pain and they include:

(a) Working to enhance posture
(b) Performing low-impact exercises, such as swimming
(c) Day to day stretching
(d) Staying active

If pain is not alleviated by oral medications or physical therapy, your physician may recommend **nerve block injections** for more efficient relief.

There are various issues to assess and decide treatment options after a confirmed scoliosis diagnosis:

(a) **Spinal maturity-** This is to check if the patient's spine is still growing and changing. The risk of worsening is lesser if the individual's bones have stopped growing. Braces are more efficient while the bones are still growing.

(b) **Location of curve-** Thoracic curve is more likely to progress than curves in other parts of the spine and this is according to some experts. In other words, a curve in the center region of the spine is more likely to get worse than a curve in the lower or upper region or section.

(c) **Extent and degree of curvature-** This is to determine how severe is the curve and how it affect the lifestyle of the patient. Larger curves are more likely to aggravate with time. S-shaped curves are typical in individuals with idiopathic scoliosis, while C-shaped curves are more common among those with neuromuscular scoliosis.

(d) **Sex-** Females have a much increased risk of progression than males.

Treatment Options

1. **Bracing-** An individual with scoliosis may be required to make use of a brace if they are still growing and the curvature is more than 25° to 40°. Braces are typically effective in patients who have not attained skeletal maturity.

   Braces won't strengthen the spine, although they can prevent the curvature from increasing. This treatment method is more efficient for cases that are detected on time. There have been advancements in brace design and the newer models fit under the arm and not around the neck. There are various types of braces available and while there is some disagreement among experts as to which type of brace is most effectual, large studies suggest that braces, when used with total compliance, successfully stop curve progression in around 80% of children with scoliosis. For maximum effectiveness, the brace should be check frequently to assure a correct and proper fit.

Individuals requiring a brace need to wear it 16 to 23 hours daily until the growth stops. The effectiveness of a brace increases with the number of hours they wear it each day. Children who wear braces can often participate in most activities and have few restrictions. If imperative, kids can take off the brace to participate in sports or other physical activities.

Physicians often suggest that children wear their braces until they attain adolescence and are no longer growing. Braces are discontinued when there are no further or continuous changes in height.

Types of bracing

(a) **Underarm/Thoracolumbosacral orthosis-** Composed of plastic and fitting close to the body, this type of brace is practically invisible under the clothes, as it fits under the arms and around the rib cage, lower back and hips. The underarm which is the most common type of brace is used in treating lower spine curves and fits around the lower region of the body.

(b) Milwaukee- This kind of brace begins at the neck and covers the whole torso, with the exception of the legs and arms. The Milwaukee brace is used for curves that the underarm brace can't solve.

2. **CASTING-** A physician may make use of plaster casting in infant with scoliosis rather than bracing to aid the infant's spine grow into a normal position. The cast attaches to the outside of the body of the infants, and they will wear it always. As most infants grow speedily, the physician will

need to change the cast frequently.

Some individuals consult or visit a **chiropractor** *to alleviate the pain and discomfort of scoliosis. Chiropractors manipulate the spine and offer alternative treatments. They maintain that realigning the spine will enhance healing and well-being.*

Chiropractic treatment *may enhance the quality of life for an individual with scoliosis. Nevertheless, it is not a cure as it does not fix the curvature of the spine. Research has not demonstrated that chiropractic manipulations have benefits for scoliosis.*

Individuals who choose to visit a chiropractor should take care to choose one who specializes in scoliosis since receiving chiropractic treatment from a non-specialist can aggravate symptoms.

Certain therapies can help in managing scoliosis pain, although they won't help in correcting the curvature itself.

Some techniques require more research but may be recommended or suggested by your physician and they include **massage, back braces, hydrotherapy, as well as electrical stimulation.**

These methods are most likely to help decrease pain and discomfort.

CHAPTER EIGHT

SURGERY FOR SCOLIOSIS

Surgery is often reserved for individuals with curves higher than 40° and if there are signs of progression. Nevertheless, speak to your physician about surgical options if you have been diagnosed with scoliosis and feel the curvature is disrupting your day to day life or causing you discomfort.

Surgery may be recommended for the following reasons and they include:

(a) **Pain-** Surgery may be required if back and leg pain from the scoliosis becomes intense and does not respond to conservative treatment.

There are a range of spinal surgical alternatives or options, and this depends on each case. Typically, surgical techniques are designated to stabilize the spine, restore balance, and ease pressure on nerves. Spine stabilization surgery connects the bones of the spine together using bone grafts and then metallic implants to hold the spine in position.

Severe scoliosis basically progresses with time, and thus your physician might recommend surgery to help straighten the curve.

Spinal fusion is the standard scoliosis surgery and in this technique or procedure, the physician connects two or more bones in your vertebrae together so they can't move independently. A bone graft, metal rods, hook, or screw is being used for this method. A bone-like material or pieces of bone are placed in between the spine (vertebrae). The ***bone graft*** comprises of bone or a material like it.

The rods help in keeping your spine in a straight position, while the screws hold them in place.

*If the scoliosis is progressing quickly at a young age, surgeons can connect one or two **expandable rods** along the spine that can adjust in length as the child grows. The rods are expanded every 3 to 6 months either with surgery or in the hospital using a remote control.*

*The **Vertebral body tethering** procedure or technique can be performed via small incisions. Screws are positioned along the outside edge of the abnormal spinal cure and a firm, flexible rod is threaded through the screws. When the cord is expanded or lengthened, the spine straightens and as the child grows, the spine may further straighten.*

Furthermore, there are some risks associated with spinal surgery and they include:

(a) Rod displacement- A rod may move from its appropriate position, making further surgery essential.

(b) Nerve damage- **Nerve damage** can occur to the nerves of the spine resulting into issues that range from moderate, such as *leg numbness, to severe, such as a loss of lower body function.*

(c) Pseudoarthritis- This is the inability of the bones to fuse or connect. It may be painful and can result into a failure of the rods since all metal will fail with exposure to persistent stress.

(d) Infection

(e) Pain

(f) Failure to heal

(g) Excessively Bleeding

In children, the two (2) main goals or objectives of surgery are to stop the curve from progressing during adulthood and to lessen spinal deformity.

Surgery is often recommended only when the spinal curve is greater than 40° and if there are signs of progression. This surgery can be performed using an **anterior approach** i.e through the front or a **posterior approach** i.e through the back and this depends on the specific cause.

Some adults who were treated as children may require revision surgery, and specifically, if they were treated 20 to 30 years ago, before major advances in spinal surgery techniques were executed. Initially, it was common to connect a long segment of the spine and when numerous vertebral segments of the spine are connected together, the remaining mobile segments assume much more of the load and the stress related with movements. Adjacent segment disease is the process in which degenerative changes occur gradually in the mobile segments above and below the spinal fusion. This can cause painful arthritis of the discs, ligaments and facet joints.

Generally, surgery in adults may be suggested or recommended when the spinal curve is greater than 50° and the patient has nerve damage to their legs and/or is experiencing bowel symptoms. Adults with degenerative scoliosis and spinal stenosis may require decompression surgery along with spinal fusion and a surgical technique from both the front and back.

A host of factors can result into increased surgical-related risks in older adults with degenerative scoliosis and these factors may include:

(a) Being a smoker
(b) Advanced age
(c) Presence of other health/medical issues.

On the general perspective, both surgery and time of recovery are expected to take more time in older adults with scoliosis.

The most commonly performed surgery for adolescent idiopathic scoliosis involves posterior spinal fusion with instrumentation and bone grafting and this is performed via the back while the patient lies on his or her stomach. During this surgery, the spine is straightened with strong metal rods, and then by spinal fusion. Spinal fusion literally involves adding a bone graft to the curved region of the spine, which in turn establishes a strong connection between two or more vertebrae.

This technique often takes several hours in children, although will typically take longer in older adults. With recent technological advances, most individuals with idiopathic scoliosis are discharged within one (1) week of surgery and do not require post-surgical bracing. Most patients are able to return back to school in two (2) to four (4) weeks post surgery and are capable of resuming all pre-surgical activities within the period of four (4) to six (6) months.

During the **anterior approach,** the patient lies on his or her side during the surgery and the surgeon makes incisions in the patient's side, punctures the lung and removes a rib in order to reach the spine. Video-assisted thorascopic (VAT) surgery provides improved visualization of the spine and is a less invasive surgery than an open technique. The anterior spinal approach possesses various potential advantages and they include:

(a) Faster patient rehabilitation
(b) Better deformity correction
(c) Enhanced spine mobilization
(d) Fusion of fewer segments

Potential disadvantages are that numerous patients need bracing for various months post surgery, and this technique has a greater risk of morbidity.

Minimally invasive surgery- Fusion can occasionally be done through smaller incisions via minimally invasive surgery. The use of advanced fluoroscopy and endoscopy has enhanced the accuracy of incisions and hardware placement, thus reducing or decreasing tissue trauma while enabling a minimally invasive surgery procedure.

Decompressive Laminectomy- The laminae (roof) of the vertebrae are removed to establish more space for the nerves and a spinal fusion with or without spinal instrumentation is usually suggested when scoliosis and spinal stenosis are present. Several devices (such as screws or rods) may be used in improving fusion and support unstable regions of the spine.

The importance of surgery should always be weighed accurately against its risks, although a great percentage of scoliosis patients benefit from surgery. Nevertheless, there is certainty that surgery will stop curve progression and symptoms in literally every individual.

CHAPTER NINE

NATURAL HOME REMEDIES FOR SCOLIOSIS

Mild scoliosis is usually managed simply with exercise, medical observation, scoliosis-specific physical therapy, and chiropractic treatment from a chiropractic scoliosis specialist. Nevertheless, for some individuals with scoliosis, yoga or pilates is also suggested or recommended to reduce their level of pain and increase flexibility.

Moderate scoliosis usually involves bracing to discontinue the spine from curving further and depending on the curvature of the spine; your physician may recommend increased medical observation or other treatment options.

As soon as the spine reaches a certain advanced curvature, and as soon as the individual with scoliosis reaches a certain age, surgery becomes the most recommended treatment alternative. Surgery to repair scoliosis can take various forms and depends on a range of factors, such as:

(a) The way your spine is shaped and how tall you are
(b) Whether or not other parts of your body have been seriously impaired by the growth of your spine.

The spine plays a vital role in the general health of an individual as well as supporting the body for posture and movement. While they follow a natural S-shaped curvature front to back, most individual spines maintain a vertical line straight up and down. Individuals living with scoliosis, nevertheless, have an abnormal curvature of the spine to the left or right and this can result into scoliosis back pain, stiffness, fatigue and a host of physical ailments resulting from posture alignment.

While some cases of scoliosis may require more drastic intervention, many individuals are capable of treating their symptoms naturally at home.

Taking care of your spine is completely crucial to your general health. Taking care of your back can have a major influence on your day to day life and if you are one of the millions of individuals living with scoliosis, finding simple ways to manage symptoms and reduce pain can drastically enhance your quality of life.

Some of the natural home remedies for scoliosis pain include:

1. **Pain relief exercises-** There are numerous exercises you can perform for scoliosis pain relief

that are excellent for your spine. These exercises are primarily focused on strengthening your core muscles for effective bodily support. Some of the **easy core strengthening activities** you can introduce into your day to day fitness include:

- Glute bridges
- Seated rotations
- Planking

Low-impact exercises such as **tai-chi, yoga, walking, running, hiking, rowing, and swimming** are usually excellent as well. You don't require a complete home gym or a gym membership to complete full body workout exercises aimed at building core strength and as a matter of fact, many of these can even be done in combination with **athlete recovery tools such as a zero gravity chair.**

Rowing helps in strengthening the back muscles, which in turn keep the spine straight. Swimming is a well-rounded exercise that helps in developing the muscles of the whole body. Nevertheless, avoid competitive swimming.

Furthermore, it is vital to consult a doctor since not all exercises are ideal for scoliosis as some may even aggravate it.

2. **Stretches-** Stretching first thing in the morning are a simple method for treating symptoms of scoliosis at home and these stretches help in loosening up the body, reducing excess pressure and tension on the spine.

   Some simple stretches for scoliosis may include:
   (a) Cat-camel stretch
   (b) Pelvic tilts

(c) Lattissimus dorsi stretch

(d) Abdominal press

These stretches are appropriate to begin your day, although they may also be vital to include as part of a pre-workout warm-up and post workout recovery routine.

3. **Heat Therapy-** Heat Therapy is another natural home remedy you may consider trying.

    Heat therapy help with:

    - Loosening muscles
    - Enhancing blood circulation for faster bodily healing
    - Maintaining a healthy spine.

Although a heating pad is an easy way to apply heat to your body, there are more effectual methods for treating scoliosis at home. Once more, zero gravity chairs may become the proper tool for scoliosis pain relief as the combined advantages of a zero *gravity recliner with heat and massage functions relieve your body.* A *heated zero gravity chair* may exemplify on the effects of the zero gravity position and massage features to relieve scoliosis back pain, keep muscles loose as well as help in living a pain-free life.

4. **Spinal decompression-** Spinal decompression therapy relieves the damages done to the spine by carefully stretching it out, alleviating spinal pressure and promoting spinal healing. The spinal decompression therapy is an effectual way to enhance your posture by repositioning the spine into the natural curve and potentially bringing about scoliosis pain relief.

   Spinal decompression is the gentle and careful stretching of the spine to ***ease lower back pain*** and promote spinal healing. As the spine is stretched back out, pressure is discharged from discs and off the nerves along the body. Spinal decompression may also be appropriate for individuals looking out for ***sciatica treatment at home.***

5. **Nutrition-** It is vital to take a balanced diet and avoid some type of unhealthy foods.

6. **Supplements and Herbal remedies-** You can take several supplements and herbs to fulfill the nutritional requirements that might cause your condition.

7. Massage and physical therapy

Coping with scoliosis can be hard for a young individual in an already complicated phase of life. Teens are bombarded with physical changes and emotional and social challenges and with the added diagnosis of scoliosis; adolescents may feel anger, insecurity, and fear.

Support group members can offer advice, relay real-life experiences and help you link with others facing similar challenges and difficulties.

CHAPTER TEN

SCOLIOSIS DIET

An unhealthy diet is more than just empty calories as **hormone and neurotransmitter imbalances** can all contribute to scoliosis progression. Still, poor nutrition by itself does not result into idiopathic scoliosis as children either have the **genetic predisposition** or they don't. Studies do connect worsening of the condition to nutritional deficiencies and a lack of healthy eating.

Researchers were able to conclude two decades ago that poor nutrition may play a role in idiopathic scoliosis and that this possibility should be examined further in humans. Nevertheless, more current studies have shown that in individuals who carry the scoliosis genes, specific nutritional imbalances can influence whether a curve develops or progresses.

While poor nutrition does not result into idiopathic scoliosis, progression can be triggered by hormone imbalances, certain mineral deficiencies or an unhealthy diet. This is as a result of the way the brain and muscles communicate with each other.

Enhancing your family's diet to support your child can decrease the risk of scoliosis progression and majority of these diet suggestions are excellent for any individual, with or without scoliosis to reduce risk of heart disease, prevent obesity and high blood pressure (hypertension).

Consuming snacks and foods that have chemical additives, calories from sugar, and preservatives can result into chronic inflammation. Inflammation is a stress response that makes the body to deliver cytokines. Progressively, this results into loss of bone. Individuals with high indicators for inflammation suffer 73% more hip fractures. It also drains your muscles and weak muscles have a much difficult time holding the spine in place.

Numerous chemical additives impoverished the bones and muscles of nutrients.

For instance,

- Salt leads to excessive mineral excretion via the kidneys.
- Sugar and soda impede the ability of the body to absorb calcium.
- Alcohol contributes to low bone mass and restricts bone formation.
- Caffeine drains calcium from bones at the rate of 6 milligrams of lost calcium for every 100 milligrams of caffeine ingested.

Numerous individuals believe that intake of low-fat dairy beverages are excellent sources of calcium, but in fact have highly reduced health benefits. Limiting citrus fruit juices is highly recommended.

Purchase organic fruits and vegetables as often as possible since non-organic foods usually have carcinogens, pesticides, neurotoxins, hormone disruptors, as well as developmental toxins connected to health tissues and disease.

Nutrition is highly beneficial for scoliosis patients for a host of reasons:

(a) There is a linkage between a neurotransmitter deficiency and the development of scoliosis and by incorporating precursors to neurotransmitters *such as amino acids* into the diet, the body can produce them naturally, which has a remarkably positive influence on the condition.

(b) Numerous scoliosis patients are unable to methylate the vitamin B12 (riboflavin) efficiently. Methylation is a crucial biological process that helps the body in producing neurotransmitters such as *serotonin and dopamine.*

(c) A healthy diet helps patients decrease the possibility they **will suffer** from chronic inflammation, which can result into a loss of bone density.

(d) Leaner patients respond more positively to treatments, specifically individuals who are adolescent patients.

Food items that are packed and loaded with sugar, salt and unhealthy fats are somewhat not good for a proper scoliosis diet.

Foods to avoid or limit

(a) Pasteurized milk/pasteurized dairy products

(b) Coffee

(c) Trans fats/hydrogenated fats

(d) Alcohol – Excess alcohol lead to decreased bone mass.

(e) White flour

(f) Soy milk and other form of soy products

(g) Artificial sweeteners such as *Splenda, Saccharin, Aspartame, Saccharin, Acesulfamine, Sucralose, Neotame, Nutrasweet, Equal, etc.*

(h) Excess salt, although moderate amount of sea salt is okay- Excessive salt can lead to loss of calcium through your urine.

(i) Greasy and fried foods- particularly those from fast food restaurants.

(j) Sugar, although stevia is an excellent substitute –Sugary drinks impede the body's ability to absorb calcium

(k) Monosodium glutamate

(l) Chocolate, although dark chocolate is ideal in limited quantities

(m) Foods comprising of corn syrup in any form (high fructose, crystallized, etc)

(n) Soda pop

(o) Packaged luncheon meats as they comprise of numerous food additives and preservatives which can lead to excessive inflammation.

(p) Fast food or other highly processed varieties of *junk* food

(q) Citrus fruits and citrus juices such as *tomato juice*

(r) Glutamic acid, sodium caseinate, and autolyzed yeast.

(s) Gelatin, caseinate

(t) Hydrolyzed vegetable protein

(u) Monopotassium glutamate, textured protein

(v) Yeast extract, hydrolyzed plant protein.

(w)Refined vegetable oils such as *canola, corn and soybean oils which are high in pro-inflammatory omega-6 fatty acids.*

(x) Refined carbohydrates and processed grain products and added sugars *found in mosr packaged snacks, condiments, bread, cereals, and canned items.*

Foods to eat and consume for scoliosis

The following food items offer excellent nutrition and **enhance the body's ability to recover successfully from scoliosis.**

(a) **Non-processed Meats-** Turkey, chicken, fish, beef, seafood (oysters), and lean meats provide crucial protein to the body. Just ensure to avoid oily or fried meats, such as those you would get at a fast food restaurant and also steer clear or avoid packaged lunch meats and pork, which comprises of preservatives and other unhealthy add ons.

(b) **Foods comprising of Calcium and Vitamin D-** Calcium is a highly essential mineral in the human body, and it is essential for scoliosis patients to introduce into their diets through supplements or whole foods. *Poppy, sesame, celery and chia seeds all comprise of high amounts of calcium.* Beans and lentils also contain calcium, as well as a host of other beneficial minerals. If you also desire healthy snacks, almonds are also great.

Vitamin D is also essential, largely due to the fact that numerous individuals do not get enough of it. Supplements are beneficial, although vitamin D can also be found in various foods, such as *mushrooms, eggs, and fish.*

(c) Water- Although it is not technically a food, water is crucial in the correct scoliosis diet. Proper hydration keeps all the body's systems in top working order as well as helps in most of the body's natural processes.

Water is also the ideal substitute for soda, coffee, alcoholic beverages and other unhealthy drinks.

(d) Vegetables and Fresh fruits-
Vegetables and fresh fruits are loaded with nutrients that are essential for the health and maintenance of the human body. They also comprise of fiber, which is something that is literally lacking from most diets. In addition, the consumption of vegetables and fresh fruits can contribute to a decreased risk of chronic disease.

Aim for variety and a minimum of 4 to 5 servings of fresh vegetables each day. 3 to 4 servings of fresh fruits each day are excellent for most individuals.

Some of the healthy vegetables and fresh fruits include:

(a) Apples

(b) Broccoli

(c) Kale

(d) Pears

(e) Peaches

(f) Celery

(g) Green beans

(h) Avocado

(i) Brussels sprouts

(j) Tomatoes

(k) Carrots

(l) Coconut

(m) Cauliflower

(n) Tofu

(o) Lentils

(p) Peas, chickpeas

(q) Leafy green vegetables

(r) Fresh non-citrus fruits.

5. High fiber foods- Plant-based foods are typically high in fiber, which is required for appropriate gut health and detoxification.

6. Anti-inflammatory herbs, spices, and teas such as *ginger, basil, oregano, thyme, turmeric, etc.*

7. Probiotic foods such as *yogurt, kombucha, kefir, kvass, or cultured veggies* help in restoring gut health and preventing inflammation.

8. Healthy fats- Healthy fats help in balancing hormones and reducing inflammation. Make use of grass-fed butter, extra virgin olive oil, coconut oil, nuts/seeds etc.

9. Bone Broth- Bone broth comprises of collagen which helps in maintaining healthy joints as well as help in treating the lining of the gut.

10. High quality protein from grass-fed animals

11. Ancient grains as well as legumes/beans.

Over-the-counter supplements for scoliosis

Tests and diagnosis have indicated that scoliosis patients have high levels of osteopontin, which modulates *bone growth* and if your child has a deficiency in selenium, it may be causing high osteopontin levels and abnormal bone growth. 200 micrograms of selenium daily can reduce osteopontin levels as it may slow or stop the risk of rapid scoliosis progression. This may be one of the supplements to steer clear of after spinal fusion.

After nutritional screening, there are some supplements to consider and they include:

1. **Probiotic-** A probiotic that promotes healthy bacteria in the intestine is beneficial for supporting digestive health.
2. **EPA-DHA Complex-** These omega-3 fatty acids play a crucial role in helping the brain function

as effective scoliosis treatment requires ***retraining the posture memory.***

3. **Collagenics-** The combination and mixture of free-form amino acids, key minerals and other nutrients help in the development of postural strength.

4. **Vitamin D3 (cholecalciferol) and K2 (menaquinones)** - Vitamin D plays a crucial role in helping the body absorb calcium and this is vital for increasing and maintaining bone density. It also helps in supporting the metabolism as well as neurological functions.

5. **Multigenics-** Vitamin supplements for scoliosis, calcium and amino acids enhance the health of a liver and a healthy liver allows the absorption of vitamins A, D, E, and K. It also

helps in producing enzymes that help in transporting nutrients.

6. **Inflavonoids-** These herbal pain relievers combine herbs such as turmeric, ginger, curcumin, vitamin C (ascorbic acid), and supplements for lower back pain and scoliosis.

7. **Magnesium-** A high percentage of patients with scoliosis appear to have deficiency of magnesium. Magnesium is essential for muscle, bone and spinal health, which is why low magnesium levels are linked to *muscle spasms/*painful muscle contractions, osteoporosis, fractures and osteopenia

8. **Essential oil** such as frankincense oil can be applied basically on the spine to relieve pain and accelerate healing.

9. **Omega-3 fish oil** is a natural anti-inflammatory that helps in decreasing pain and accelerating healing.

Patients can improve the effectiveness of treatment with diet and the best supplements for scoliosis.

CHAPTER ELEVEN

EXERCISES AND STRETCHING EXERCISES FOR SCOLIOSIS

Exercise is helpful for scoliosis patients when used alone or in combination with other treatments *such as bracing.*

Exercise can help in building and maintaining core strength to support the spine and this is vital since stronger muscles help in stabilizing the spine.

Some of the benefits of therapeutic exercises may include:

(a) Decrease symptoms such as *pain, fatigue, and trunk symptoms.*

(b) Stop scoliosis progression

(c) Improve flexibility as well as mobility

(d) Prevent instability as a result of spinal degeneration

(e) Enhance lung function and breathing

(f) Enhance muscular strength as well as endurance.

(g) Prevent or stop worsening spinal curvature

(h) Enhance mood and confidence

The most effective scoliosis treatment exercises combine strengthening and stretching. Strengthening exercises help in building muscle strength and endurance in your core to retard or slow the progression of the spinal curve and decrease scoliosis-associated pain as well as discomfort. Stretching exercises boost flexibility to decrease spine rigidity and increase range of motion.

Exercises for Children with scoliosis

Most children with scoliosis do not have scoliosis-associated pain. Most exercises for children with scoliosis focus on neuromuscular control to maintain and support the trunk.

Some of the exercises for children with scoliosis may include:

(a) Prone plank
(b) Pelvic tilts
(c) Cat-camel
(d) Leg lifts while lying on the back
(e) Double leg abdominal press as well as bird-dog stretches.

Exercises for teenagers with scoliosis

Teenagers with adolescent idiopathic scoliosis may experience:

- Gait deviations
- Decreased flexibility
- Altered posture
- Muscular imbalance

Nevertheless, if their scoliosis is visibly recognizable, some teenagers may struggle with body image, posture, and low-self esteem.

Back and core strengthening exercises for teens integrate movements that invigorate and build muscles in the shoulders and back while keeping the spine in a neutral position.

Some of the exercises for teenagers with scoliosis may include:

(a) Plank
(b) Sitting rotation stretch
(c) Wall stands
(d) Pelvic tilts as well as ketttlebell suitcase deadlift.

Low-impact exercises such as Pilates, yoga, and tai-chi can help in boosting trunk flexibility and range of motion. Some scoliosis exercise programs, such as the **Schroth method,** *may help teenagers in decreasing the* *magnitude and progression of their spinal curve.*

Exercises for Adults with scoliosis

Adults who did not develop scoliosis in adolescence are most usually diagnosed with ***degenerative scoliosis.***

Scoliosis exercise programs for adults originally focus on enhancing flexibility as well as range of motion to resolve spinal rigidity.

Stretches for adults with scoliosis may include:

(a) Child's pose
(b) Cat/cow
(c) Seated twist and seated butterfly stretch
(d) Kneeling hip flexor stretch

As soon as flexibility is enhanced, strength exercises can be integrated to help stabilize the spine and reduce pain and discomfort.

Exercises that focus on building core strength to support the spine are highly suggested and recommended to help adults address degenerative scoliosis.

Strength exercises for adults with scoliosis may include:

(a) Glute bridges
(b) Plank
(c) Pelvic tilt
(d) Bird dog
(e) Hip thrusts
(f) Arm and leg raises
(g) Strength training on resistance machines as well as bird dog.

Exercises for seniors with scoliosis

About 68% of adults over the age of 65 may develop or have scoliosis. In older adults, scoliosis may be as a result of slow degeneration of spinal discs, which makes the spine tip to one side. Degenerative scoliosis in older adults can result into back and leg pain that reduces mobility.

Exercises for seniors originally focus on targeted stretching to decrease spinal tension and enhance flexibility. As soon as flexibility increases, core exercises for scoliosis can be incorporated to build strength and boost balance and posture. Older adults are at a greater risk of falls, and thus balance is particularly vital.

Some of the exercises for seniors with scoliosis may include:

(a) Child's pose
(b) Lying hip stretch
(c) Pilates
(d) Yoga
(e) Tai chi
(f) Standing on one leg
(g) Sitting on an exercise ball

(h) Overhead stretch as well as wall stretch

Schroth Method

The schroth which is a scoliosis-specific exercise program takes a 3-dimensional approach to resolve all three spinal anatomical planes which are the *sagittal plane, transverse plane, and the frontal plane.*

Schroth method helps in:

(a) Increasing patient postural awareness

(b) Enhancing breathing and lung capacity

(c) Building muscle strength and endurance

(d) Boosting and improving posture

(e) Reducing pain caused by muscle imbalance

(f) Preventing or stopping curve progression

Some of the schroth method exercise programs may include:

(a) Posture correction procedures
(b) *Working with props such as exercise bands, therapy balls, and poles.*
(c) Low-impact exercises in sitting, standing, and lying down positions.
(d) Rotational angular breathing exercises

Patients treated with this method are advised to integrate the techniques they learn while engaging in day to day activities such as sitting, standing, and walking.

Exercises and stretching exercises for scoliosis

Exercises for scoliosis help in increasing core strength, enhancing your posture as well as strengthening the muscles in your lower back.

In mild cases, individuals treating their scoliosis with specific exercises and stretches *can prevent* the need for surgery, although an individual with scoliosis should consult a physician before performing stretches and exercises for scoliosis.

Individuals with lumbar scoliosis should focus on exercising their lower back. On the contrary, individuals with thoracic scoliosis should focus more on exercising their thoracic spine as well as upper back.

Some of the stretches and exercises that are highly recommended may include:

(a) Arm and Leg Raises- An individual can strengthen their lower back with arm and leg raises.

Directions

- Lie on your front with your forehead to the ground and extend your arms straight over your head with your palms or fists on the ground.
- Keep both legs straight and raise your arms and legs off the ground.
- Hold for a complete breath, and then lower your arms and legs back down.
- Iterate 15 times.

(b) Cat-cow- The Cat-cow is type of *yoga* pose which can help in keeping the spine flexible and pain-free.

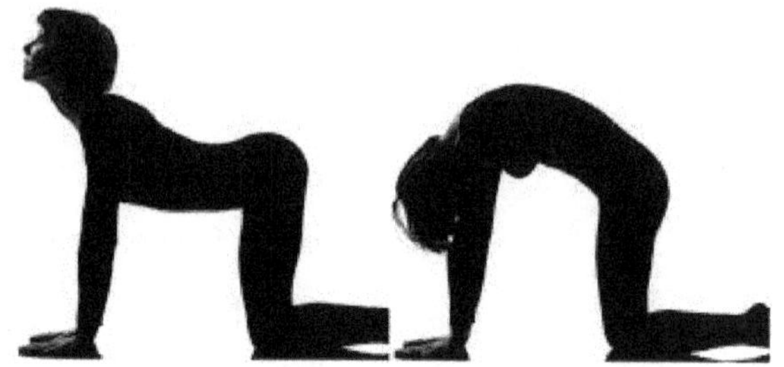

Directions

- Start on your hands and knees, making sure your back is level and your head and neck are comfortable.
- Inspire or inhale deeply while drawing your abdominal muscles in and up, arching your back.
- Expire or exhale while releasing your abdominal muscles, dropping your back, allowing your belly fall, and lifting your head toward the ceiling.
- Perform 2 sets of 10.

(c) Latissimus dorsi stretch- The Latissimus dorsi stretch focuses on the latissiumus dorsi which is the largest muscle in the upper body of the human.

Directions

- Stand with good posture in a neutral position and keep your feet shoulder-width apart with your knees very slightly bent.
- Reaching over your head with both hands, grab the right wrist with the left hand and bend slightly toward the right side until you feel a stretch in your left side of your body.
- Hold for one to two breaths, and then carefully pull with the

left hand to straighten
and return to the initial
position.

- Iterate on the opposite side
- Perform 5 to 10 repetitions on each side for better posture.

(d) Abdominal press- Firm abdominal muscles can help in taking some pressure off of the back muscles and enhance good posture.

Directions

- With your feet flat on the ground and your knees bent, lie on your back and keep the back in a neutral, tension-free position.
- Raise both feet off of the floor until your thighs and feet form a 90°

angle, and your knees are above the hips.

- Use your hands to push your knees away while concurrently pulling your knees toward your hands with your abdominal muscles. This is a static exercise, which entails that the legs and arms should not move when pressing.
- Hold for three complete breaths, relax and perform 2 sets of 10.

(e) Sitting rotation stretch- This can help in enhancing your flexibility, which in turn decrease some of the back pain you may be experiencing.

Directions

- Sit on the floor or an exercise mat and cross

your right leg over the left.

- Place the sole of the right leg on the floor and place your right arm behind you as a form of support.
- Twist your torso towards the right leg and extend your left arm so the elbow presses against the knee.
- Look over your right shoulder to deepen the stretch and hold for as long as recommended by your personal trainer.

(f) Kettlebell Suitcase Deadlift- This exercise helps in increasing the strength of the convex side of the spine, which may help in alleviating some of your back pain.

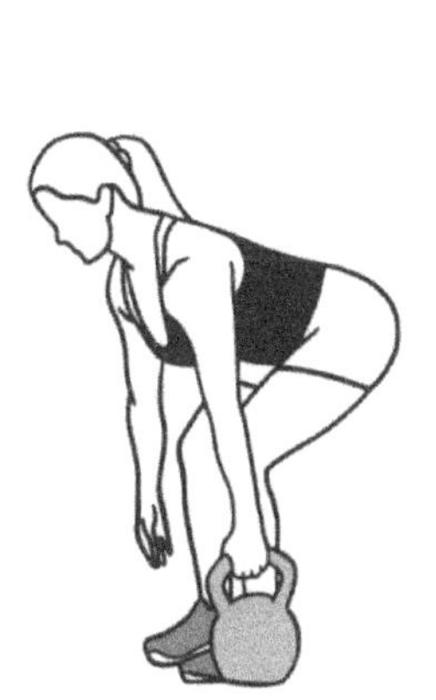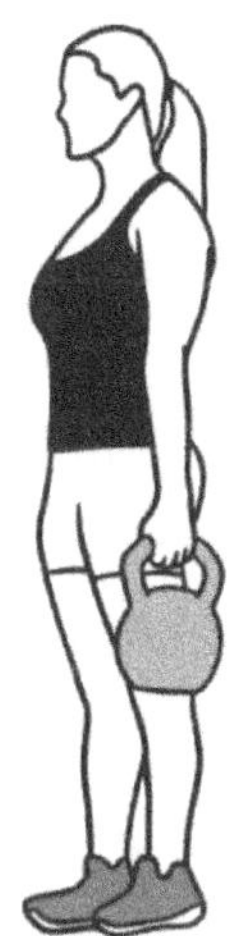

Directions

- Select a kettlebell weight that you can lift with one hand and stand up straight with your feet hip-width apart.

- Position the kettlebell on the outside of your right foot.

- Hinge at the hips, bending your knees and keeping your

spine straight, grab the kettlebell and stand up with a neutral spine to pick it up.

- Iterate as directed.

(g) Plank- The plank which is an easy but effective exercise for strengthening your core muscle is divided into four (4) different levels.

1st level- Elbows and Knees

- Lying on your stomach, raise your torso by resting on your elbows, ensuring your shoulders and elbows are in line.
- Your forearms should be completely on the ground in front of you, parallel to each other, and your elbow at about 90° angle.

- With your knees on the ground, lift your abs and ensure you are not bending your hips or arching your back.

2nd Step- Hands and Knees

- Get on your hands and knees and ensure your wrists are directly beneath your shoulders.
- Your knees should not be in line with your hips but behind them with your torso in a straight line from shoulders to knees.
- Hold as long as recommended.

3rd step- Elbows and feet

- Get on your hands and knees and extend your legs behind you with toes flexed.
- Place your elbows on the ground directly beneath your shoulders and with your body in a straight line from your shoulders to your toes, hold for as long as recommended.

4th step- Hands and feet

- Get on your hands and knees and extend your legs behind you with toes flexed.
- Ensure your body is in one line from shoulders to toes and hold for as long as you can or as recommended.

(h) Bird-dog

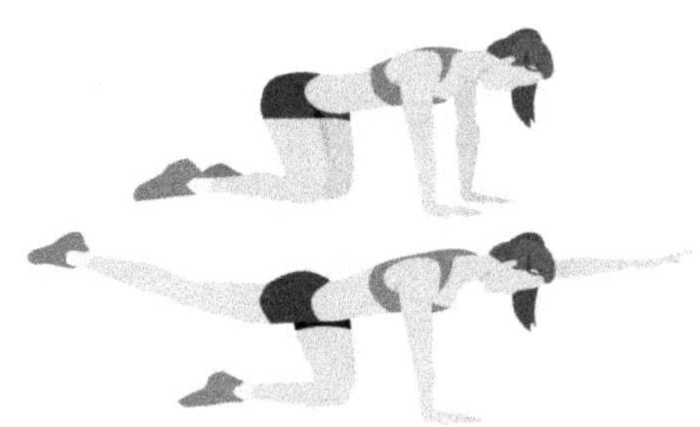

Directions

- Start and get on your hands and knees with a straight back and place your hands directly under your shoulders with your knees under your hips.

- Extend one arm straight out and forward while extending the opposite leg straight back, and then

breathe normally and hold
for around 5 seconds.

- Iterate with the opposite
  arm and leg.
- Perform 10 to 15
  repetitions on each side.

(i) Pelvic tilts- This will help in
stretching tight muscles in the
hips and lower back.

Directions

- With your knees bent and
  your feet flat on the floor,
  lie on your back and
  tighten your stomach
  muscles while flattening
  your back toward the
  floor.
- Hold for 5 seconds while
  breathing normally,
  release and perform 2 sets
  of 10 to continue building
  your lower back muscles.

(j) Performing good posture- Excellent posture can decrease pain and muscle tension. Several times each day, an individual can realign their body to help in learning how to stand with an excellent posture naturally.

Directions

- Drop your shoulders down and back and position your ears over your shoulders.
- Gently tuck your chin in, so it is not jutting forward or very far down.
- Draw the stomach in slightly and unlock, or bend the knees slightly.

Keep your back straight and the ears over your shoulders when sitting. An individual should keep his or her legs in a neutral position and not crossed as this can help in scanning the body for signs of tension.

What to avoid

Some exercises and activities can aggravate scoliosis symptoms or increase the risk of secondary injuries. Individuals with should steer clear or avoid:

(a) Playing football and other high contact sports as they can be dangerous for individuals with scoliosis.

(b) Exposing the spine to iterated impacts from jumping or running. Common culprits may include:

- Horseback riding
- Trampolines
- Long-distance running on hard surfaces.

(c) Keeping their neck bent forward with their head facing downward, such as when making use of smart phone.

(d) Repeatedly extending the torso which can take place or occur in certain *yoga positions, gymnastic maneuvers as well as ballet steps.*

CONCLUSION

Scoliosis which is most usually diagnosed in adolescents is a sideway curvature or an abnormal lateral curvature of the spine (backbone). There is a natural forward-and-backward curve to the spine or a sideways C- or S- shaped curve in the spine.

The **normal curves** of the spine occur at the *cervical, thoracic and lumbar regions* in the supposed *"sagittal"* plane.

THE END.